Jeff Smith

THE BETTER
SLEEP SOLUTION

Unlocking the Secrets to Restful Nights

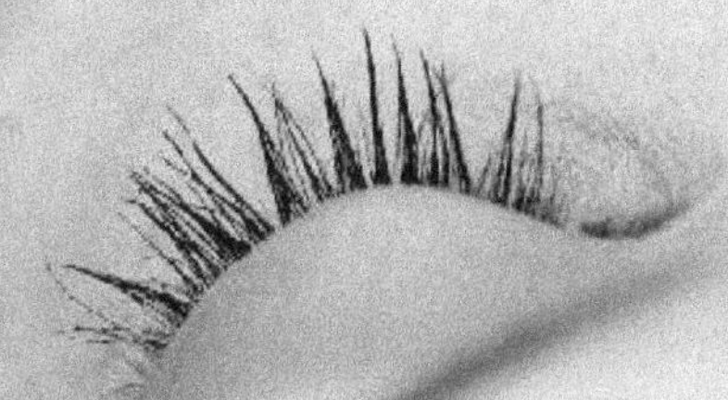

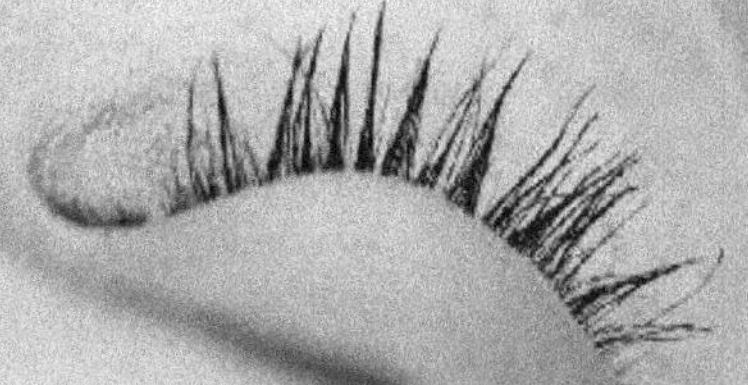

Published September 2023

Copyright Disruptive Brands LLC

www.SleepZM.com

Foreword

Welcome to "The Better Sleep Solution: Unlocking the Secrets to Restful Nights." This book is dedicated to helping Sleep ZM customers aged 18-80 discover the keys to sleeping better and experiencing the rejuvenating benefits of a good night's rest.

Whether you struggle with occasional sleeplessness or have been battling chronic insomnia for years, this book aims to provide you with practical strategies and insightsto improve your sleep quality.

Before we delve into the specific techniques and solutions, it's important to note thatthis book outline is not set in stone. The author recognizes that sleep is a complex and deeply personal experience, and what works for one person may not work for another. Therefore, feel free to adapt and modify the suggestions provided here to suit your personal preferences and unique circumstances. The goal is to find a sleep routine that works best for you.

In this book, we will explore a wide range of topics related to sleep, including the science behind sleep, common sleep disorders, and the impact of lifestyle factors on sleep quality. We will also provide practical tips and strategies to improve your sleep hygiene, create a sleep-friendly environment, and promote relaxation before bedtime.

Additionally, we will delve into the role of nutrition, exercise, and technology in sleep quality, as well as discuss the potential benefits of alternative therapies such as meditation, aromatherapy, and herbal remedies. The aim is to provide you with a comprehensive understanding of the factors that influence sleep and empower you to make informed choices that will lead to better sleep.

Remember, this book is merely a guide, and the real magic happens when you implement the strategies and techniques in your own life. So, let's embark on this journey together and unlock the secrets to restful nights, one chapter at a time.

Sweet dreams await! If you'd like to learn more about Blue Light Blocking Glasses, please go to www.sleepzm.com or search for "Sleep ZM blue light glasses" on Amazon.

TABLE OF CONTENT

Title: The Sleep Solution: Unlocking the Secrets to Restful Nights

Introduction:

Welcome to "The Sleep Solution: Unlocking the Secrets to Restful Nights." In this subchapter, we will delve into the secrets of achieving a restful night's sleep. Whether you struggle with occasional sleeplessness or chronic insomnia, this chapter will provide you with practical tips and strategies to help you sleep better. Regardless of your age, from 18 to 80, the information shared here will benefit adults of all walks oflife.

Understanding the Importance of Quality Sleep:

Sleep is not just a luxury; it is a vital aspect of our overall well-being. Adequate sleep is crucial for maintaining physical health, mental clarity, emotional balance, and productivity. Unfortunately, many adults find it difficult to achieve restorative sleepdue to various factors such as stress, poor sleep habits, or underlying health conditions. However, with the right knowledge and tools, you can unlock the secretsto restful nights.

Creating a Sleep-Inducing Environment:

One of the key factors in achieving quality sleep is creating a sleep-inducing environment. We will explore how to optimize your bedroom for sleep, including factors such as temperature, lighting, and noise. Additionally, we will discuss the importance of investing in a comfortable mattress, pillows, and bedding to enhance your sleep experience.

Establishing Healthy Sleep Habits:

Developing consistent sleep habits is essential for improving your sleep quality. We will provide practical tips on establishing a regular sleep schedule, incorporating relaxation techniques before bed, and avoiding stimulants that can hinder sleep. Moreover, we will address the impact of technology on sleep and how to create a healthy digital bedtime routine.

Managing Stress and Relaxation Techniques:

Stress and anxiety can significantly impact your ability to sleep well. We will reveal effective stress management techniques and relaxation strategies to calm your mind and prepare your body for a restful night's sleep. From deep breathing exercises to meditation, you will discover techniques that can help you unwind and promote better sleep.

Addressing Common Sleep Disorders:

Lastly, we will touch upon common sleep disorders that affect many adults, such as insomnia, sleep apnea, and restless leg syndrome. Understanding these disorders, their symptoms, and available treatment options will empower you to seek appropriate help if needed.

The Better Sleep Solution: Unlocking the Secrets to Restful Nights

Conclusion:

In this subchapter of "The Sleep Solution: Unlocking the Secrets to Restful Nights," we have explored various aspects of sleep and provided you with valuable insights and techniques to improve your sleep quality. By implementing the tips and strategies discussed here, you will be on your way to unlocking the secrets to restful nights andenjoying the numerous benefits of a good night's sleep. Remember, it is never too late to prioritize your sleep and take control of your well-being.

Chapter 1: Understanding the Importance of Sleep

The Science Behind Sleep

Understanding the science behind sleep is crucial for anyone looking to improve their sleep quality. In this subchapter, we will delve into the fascinating world of sleep and uncover the secrets to restful nights. Whether you're a young adult seeking better sleep or an older individual struggling with insomnia, this information will beinvaluable for you. Sleep is a complex biological process that involves various stages and cycles. It is regulated by our internal body clock, known as the circadian rhythm. This internal clock dictates our sleep-wake cycle, ensuring that we feel sleepy at night and alert during the day. However, modern lifestyles and external factors can disrupt this natural rhythm, leading to sleep disturbances.

One fundamental aspect of sleep is the different stages it encompasses. These stages can be divided into two main categories: non-REM (rapid eye movement) sleep and REM sleep. Non-REM sleep is further divided into three stages: N1, N2, and N3. N1 is a light sleep stage, N2 is a deeper sleep stage, and N3 is the deepest sleep stage, also known as slow-wave sleep (SWS). REM sleep is the stage where most dreaming occurs, and it is associated with cognitive function and memory consolidation.

During sleep, our body undergoes various physiological changes. Our heart rate and blood pressure decrease, allowing our body to rest and recover. The brain also plays a crucial role in sleep, with different regions becoming active or inactive depending onthe sleep stage. Sleep is essential for our physical and mental health, as it enhances memory, promotes learning, boosts creativity, and strengthens the immune system.

To improve sleep quality, it is vital to establish healthy sleep habits. This includes maintaining a consistent sleep schedule, creating a relaxing bedtime routine, and optimizing the sleep environment. Avoiding stimulants like caffeine and electronicdevices before bed is also crucial.

Understanding the science behind sleep empowers us to take control of our sleep health. By implementing evidence-based strategies, we can overcome sleep challenges and unlock the secrets to restful nights. In the upcoming chapters, we will explore specific techniques and solutions tailored to different age groups, addressing the unique sleep needs of adults ranging from 18 to 80 years old.

Remember, quality sleep is not a luxury but a necessity for leading a healthy and fulfilling life. So, let's dive deeper into the science behind sleep and unlock the secrets to better sleep for all.

The Impact of Sleep Deprivation

Sleep is a vital part of our lives, yet many adults struggle to get the restful nights they need. In today's fast-paced world, it's not uncommon for people to sacrifice sleep in favor of work, socializing, or other activities. However, what they fail to realize is the profound impact that sleep deprivation can have on their overall well-being.

Sleep deprivation, defined as not getting enough sleep over an extended period, can lead to a host of negative consequences. Firstly, it impairs cognitive function and memory. When you don't get enough sleep, your brain struggles to process information efficiently, affecting your ability to concentrate, make decisions, and recall important details. This can have a detrimental effect on your work performance, academic success, and overall productivity.

Furthermore, sleep deprivation weakens the immune system, making you more susceptible to illnesses and infections. Adequate sleep is crucial for the body to repair and rejuvenate itself. When you consistently lack sleep, your immune system becomes compromised, leaving you more vulnerable to common illnesses like colds and flu. In the long run, chronic sleep deprivation can even increase the risk of developing chronic diseases such as diabetes, heart disease, and obesity.

Sleep deprivation also impacts our emotional well-being. Lack of sleep can lead to increased irritability, mood swings, and difficulty managing stress. It can exacerbate symptoms of anxiety and depression, making it harder to maintain a positive and balanced mental state. Not only does this affect your personal relationships and quality of life, but it can also contribute to the development of mental health disorders.

Moreover, sleep deprivation has a significant effect on physical health. It increases the risk of accidents and injuries due to decreased alertness and impaired coordination. Additionally, it disrupts hormone regulation, leading to weight gain, increased appetite, and a higher likelihood of developing metabolic disorders.

In conclusion, sleep deprivation is a serious issue with far-reaching consequences. It affects our cognitive abilities, weakens the immune system, hampers emotional well- being, and poses risks to our physical health. Recognizing the importance of sleep and prioritizing it in our daily lives is essential for better overall health and well-being. By understanding the impact of sleep deprivation, we can take steps to improve our sleep habits and unlock the secrets to restful nights.

Common Sleep Disorders

In this subchapter, we will explore some of the most prevalent sleep disorders that can affect adults of all ages. Understanding these disorders is crucial for anyone looking to improve their sleep quality and overall well-being. By identifying the signsand symptoms, you can take proactive steps to address and manage these conditions.

The Better Sleep Solution: Unlocking the Secrets to Restful Nights

Insomnia is perhaps the most widely recognized sleep disorder. It is characterized by difficulty falling asleep, staying asleep, or experiencing non-restorative sleep.

Insomnia can be caused by various factors, including stress, anxiety, depression, medications, or certain medical conditions. We will delve into the underlying causes and effective strategies to overcome insomnia.

Another common sleep disorder is sleep apnea, which affects millions of individuals worldwide. Sleep apnea causes interruptions in breathing during sleep, leading to frequent awakenings and disruptions in the sleep cycle. This disorder can have severe consequences on overall health, including increased risk of heart disease and stroke. We will discuss the different types of sleep apnea, symptoms to watch out for, and available treatment options.

Restless Legs Syndrome (RLS) is a neurological disorder that causes an irresistible urge to move the legs, often accompanied by uncomfortable sensations in the limbs. RLS is known to disrupt sleep patterns as it typically worsens during periods of rest.

We will explore the causes, triggers, and management techniques to alleviate the symptoms of RLS.

Narcolepsy is a chronic neurological disorder characterized by excessive daytime sleepiness and sudden sleep attacks. People with narcolepsy often experience uncontrollable sleep episodes, which can be dangerous in certain situations. We will discuss the symptoms, diagnosis, and treatment options available for individuals living with narcolepsy.

Lastly, we will touch upon sleepwalking and night terrors, which are more common in children but can persist into adulthood. These disorders involve abnormal behaviors during sleep, such as walking, talking, or experiencing intense fear or terror. We will explore the factors contributing to these disorders and suggestions for managing them effectively.

By familiarizing ourselves with these common sleep disorders, we can better recognize the signs and seek appropriate help when needed. Remember, quality sleep is essential for overall health and well-being. In the following chapters, we will take a closer look at specific strategies and solutions to help you overcome these sleep disorders and unlock the secrets to restful nights.

Chapter 2: Assessing Your Sleep Patterns

Keeping a Sleep Diary

One of the most effective tools for improving your sleep quality is keeping a sleep diary. This simple yet powerful technique can provide valuable insights into your sleep patterns, helping you identify any underlying issues and find solutions to sleep better. In this subchapter, we will explore the importance of keeping a sleep diary and provide you with practical tips on how to get started.

Why Keep a Sleep Diary?

A sleep diary serves as a record of your sleep habits, allowing you to track various factors that may impact your sleep quality. By consistently documenting information such as bedtime, wake-up time, sleep duration, and sleep quality, you can begin to identify patterns and trends that may be affecting your ability to get a restful night'ssleep.

Moreover, a sleep diary can help you pinpoint potential triggers for sleep disturbances, such as caffeine intake, exercise routines, or stress levels. By understanding these factors, you can make informed decisions and adjustments to improve your sleep hygiene.

Getting Started with a Sleep Diary

The Better Sleep Solution: Unlocking the Secrets to Restful Nights

To begin keeping a sleep diary, you'll need a notebook or use a sleep tracking app on your smartphone. Here are some key elements to include in your sleep diary:

1. Bedtime routine: Record your pre-sleep rituals, including activities like reading, taking a warm bath, or meditating. This will help you identify relaxing habits that contribute to better sleep.

2. Sleep environment: Note the conditions of your bedroom, such as noise levels,temperature, and lighting. This information will help you optimize your sleep environment to enhance sleep quality.

3. Sleep duration: Record the time you go to bed and wake up, as well as any awakenings during the night. This will provide insights into your sleep duration andany disruptions that may be occurring.

4. Sleep quality: Rate your sleep quality on a scale of 1 to 10, with 10 being the highest. This subjective assessment will help you track improvements or setbacks inyour sleep over time.

5. Daily factors: Document any factors that may impact your sleep, such as caffeine or alcohol consumption, exercise, stress levels, or medications taken. This will allow you to identify potential triggers for sleep disturbances.

Analyzing and Making Changes

Once you have gathered enough data in your sleep diary, review it periodically to identify patterns and trends related to your sleep quality. Look for any recurring factors that may be negatively impacting your sleep and consider making changes accordingly. For instance, if you notice that consuming caffeine late in the day affects your ability to fall asleep, consider cutting back on your intake or avoiding italtogether in the evening.

Keeping a sleep diary is an essential step towards understanding your sleep patterns and making informed decisions to improve your sleep quality. By diligently tracking your sleep habits and making necessary adjustments, you can unlock the secrets to restful nights and wake up feeling refreshed and rejuvenated.

Identifying Sleep Disruptors

In our fast-paced and demanding lives, getting a good night's sleep has become increasingly elusive. Many of us find ourselves tossing and turning, unable to fall asleep or waking up multiple times throughout the night. The consequences of poor sleep can be far-reaching, affecting our mood, productivity, and overall well-being. However, before we can find effective solutions to improve our sleep, we must first identify the sleep disruptors that may be lurking in our daily routines.

Stress, one of the most common sleep disruptors, affects people of all ages. Whetherit stems from work, relationships, or other sources, stress can wreak havoc on our ability to fall and stay asleep. Learning stress management techniques, such as meditation or deep breathing exercises, can help alleviate some of the tension thatkeeps us awake at night.

Another sleep disruptor often overlooked is our exposure to electronic devices beforebedtime. The blue light emitted by smartphones, tablets, and laptops can interfere with our body's natural sleep-wake cycle. To counteract this, it is crucial to establish a technology-free zone at least an hour before bed. Instead, engage in relaxing activities such as reading a book, taking a warm bath, or practicing gentle stretching exercises.

Caffeine, a widely consumed stimulant, is another sleep disruptor that can hinder ourability to fall asleep. To ensure a restful night, it is recommended to limit caffeine intake, especially in the afternoon and evenings. Instead, opt for herbal teas or decaffeinated alternatives that promote relaxation.

Creating a sleep-friendly environment is also essential for a restful night. Factors such as excessive noise, uncomfortable bedding, or a room that is too warm or too cold can all disrupt our sleep. Investing in earplugs, comfortable pillows, and regulating the temperature in our bedroom can greatly improve the quality of our sleep.

Furthermore, it is important to establish a consistent sleep schedule. Our bodies thrive on routine, and irregular sleep patterns can throw off our internal clock. Set a regular bedtime and wake-up time, even on weekends, to help regulate your body's natural sleep-wake cycle.

Finally, it is crucial to address any underlying medical conditions that may be contributing to poor sleep. Conditions such as sleep apnea, restless leg syndrome, or chronic pain can significantly impact our ability to get a good night's rest. Seeking medical advice and treatment options can make a world of difference in improving sleep quality.

By identifying and addressing these sleep disruptors, adults of all ages can take significant steps towards achieving restful nights. Remember, a good night's sleep is not a luxury but a necessity for our overall health and well-being. So, let's prioritize our sleep, make positive changes, and unlock the secrets to better nights.

Understanding Your Sleep Needs

In order to unlock the secrets to restful nights, it is crucial to understand your individual sleep needs. We are all unique individuals with different lifestyles, schedules, and responsibilities, and therefore our sleep requirements may vary. This subchapter aims to guide adults aged 18-80 on how to assess and meet their specific sleep needs, enabling them to achieve better sleep quality.

The first step towards understanding your sleep needs is to determine the optimal duration of sleep for your body. While the general recommendation is around 7-9 hours of sleep per night for adults, it is important to recognize that some individuals may require slightly more or less sleep. Consider factors such as your age, health condition, and daily activity levels to gauge your ideal sleep duration.

Next, it is essential to establish a consistent sleep schedule. Our bodies thrive on routine, and maintaining a regular sleep-wake cycle helps synchronize our internal clock, known as the circadian rhythm. Try to go to bed and wake up at the same timeevery day, even on weekends, to promote a more restful sleep.

Another aspect to consider is the quality of your sleep environment. Create a sleep- friendly space by ensuring your bedroom is dark, quiet, and cool. Invest in a comfortable mattress and pillows that provide adequate support for your body.

Additionally, minimize distractions such as electronic devices and excessive noise, asthey can disrupt your sleep.

Understanding your sleep needs also involves evaluating your sleep habits and lifestyle choices. Avoid consuming stimulants like caffeine and nicotine close to bedtime, as they can interfere with falling asleep. Engaging in regular exercise canhelp improve sleep quality, but avoid vigorous workouts within a few hours of bedtime, as they can energize your body and make it harder to wind down.

Lastly, pay attention to any signs of sleep disorders or conditions that may be affecting your sleep quality. If you frequently experience difficulties falling or staying asleep, loud snoring, or excessive daytime sleepiness, it may be beneficial to consult a healthcare professional for further evaluation and guidance.

By understanding your sleep needs and implementing strategies tailored to your lifestyle, you can optimize the quality of your sleep and unlock the secrets to restful nights. Remember, sleep is not a luxury but a necessity for overall well-being, and investing in better sleep habits will have far-reaching benefits in your daily life.

Chapter 3: Creating a Sleep-Conducive Environment

Optimizing Your Bedroom Setup

Creating an optimal sleep environment is crucial for achieving restful nights and waking up refreshed and rejuvenated. Your bedroom should be a sanctuary dedicated to promoting deep, uninterrupted sleep. In this subchapter, we will explore the various ways you can optimize your bedroom setup to enhance your sleep quality and improve your overall well-being.

First and foremost, let's talk about the importance of a comfortable mattress and pillows. Investing in a high-quality mattress that suits your sleeping preferences and provides adequate support is essential. Similarly, choosing pillows that align with your preferred sleeping position can help alleviate any discomfort or pain you may experience during the night.

Lighting plays a significant role in regulating your sleep-wake cycle. To create a sleep-friendly environment, consider using blackout curtains or blinds to block out any external light sources that might disrupt your sleep. Additionally, opt for warm, dimmable lights in your bedroom to promote relaxation and signal to your body thatit's time to wind down.

Temperature control is another crucial aspect of optimizing your bedroom setup. Research suggests that a cooler room temperature promotes better sleep. Set yourthermostat to a comfortable, cool temperature, usually around 65-68 degrees Fahrenheit, to create an ideal sleep environment. If necessary, use fans or air conditioning to help regulate the temperature.

Decluttering your bedroom can have a significant impact on your sleep quality. Acluttered space can lead to increased stress levels, making it harder to relax and unwind. Take the time to organize your belongings and create a clean and peaceful atmosphere in your bedroom. Consider incorporating storage solutions that keep yourspace tidy and free from distractions.

Minimizing noise disturbances is crucial for achieving restful sleep. Earplugs or a white noise machine can help drown out any unwanted sounds, such as traffic or loud neighbors. You may also consider using a sleep mask to block out any light and furtherenhance your sleep quality.

Finally, it's important to create a technology-free zone in your bedroom. The blue light emitted by electronic devices can interfere with your sleep hormone production, making it harder to fall asleep. Keep your bedroom free from smartphones, tablets, and laptops, and establish a pre-sleep routine that involves disconnecting from screens at least an hour before bedtime.

By implementing these strategies and optimizing your bedroom setup, you can create an environment that promotes deep, restorative sleep. Remember, a well-rested mind and body are essential for overall health and well-being, so prioritize creating a sleep-friendly oasis in your bedroom.

The Better Sleep Solution: Unlocking the Secrets to Restful Nights

Choosing the Right Mattress and Pillows

Getting a good night's sleep is essential for our overall health and well-being. One of the key factors that contribute to a restful slumber is the quality of our mattress and pillows. In this subchapter, we will explore the importance of choosing the right mattress and pillows and provide you with some valuable tips to help you sleep better.

When it comes to selecting a mattress, there are a few factors to consider. First and foremost, you need to determine the level of firmness that suits your body type and sleeping position. Side sleepers may benefit from a softer mattress that provides better pressure relief for their hips and shoulders, while back and stomach sleepers generally prefer a firmer mattress that offers more support to maintain proper spinal alignment.

Additionally, it is crucial to consider the material of the mattress. Memory foam mattresses are known for their ability to contour to your body, relieving pressure points and ensuring a comfortable sleep. On the other hand, innerspring mattressesare known for their breathability and support, making them a suitable choice for individuals who tend to sleep hot.

Equally important are the pillows we rest our heads on. A pillow that is too firm or toosoft can lead to neck pain and discomfort, ultimately impacting the quality of sleep. There is no one-size-fits-all pillow, as the ideal pillow will vary based on personal preferences and sleep position. Back sleepers generally benefit from a medium-firm pillow that supports the natural curve of their neck, while side sleepers may find a firmer, thicker pillow more comfortable. Stomach sleepers, however, typically require a softer, flatter pillow to prevent strain on the neck.

To ensure you make the right choice, it is advisable to test out different mattresses and pillows before making a purchase. Take advantage of mattress and pillow trials offered by retailers, and don't hesitate to spend some time lying down on them to assess comfort and support.

Remember, investing in a high-quality mattress and pillows is an investment in your sleep quality and overall health. By choosing the right mattress and pillows tailored to your needs, you can significantly enhance your sleep experience and wake up feeling refreshed and rejuvenated.

In summary, when selecting a mattress and pillows, consider factors such as firmness, material, and your sleeping position. Test out different options before making a decision, and prioritize your comfort and support. By choosing the right mattress and pillows, you will be well on your way to unlocking the secrets to restful nights and enjoying the benefits of a good night's sleep.

Controlling Noise and Light Levels

In our modern, fast-paced world, it seems like silence and darkness have become rare commodities. As a result, our sleep quality suffers, leaving us tired, irritable, and unable to function at our best. If you're one of the millions of adults struggling to get a good night's sleep, it's time to take control of the noise and light levels in your sleep environment. In this subchapter, we will explore effective strategies to help you create a peaceful and restful space, ensuring that you can finally unlock the secrets to restful nights.

First and foremost, let's address the issue of noise. Unwanted sounds can be incredibly disruptive to our sleep patterns, causing us to wake up frequently or preventing us from falling asleep in the first place. To combat this, consider investing in earplugs or soundproof curtains to muffle external noises. If you live in a particularly noisy area, a white noise machine can be a game-changer, drowning out the disturbances and lulling you into a deep slumber.

Next, let's talk about light levels. Our bodies are naturally programmed to sleep when it's dark, so any form of light in your bedroom can interfere with your circadian

rhythm. Start by eliminating all sources of artificial light, such as electronics or LED displays. Consider using blackout curtains or an eye mask to create a pitch-dark

environment that signals your brain that it's time to sleep. If you're a light sleeper, even small amounts of light can disrupt your rest, so be diligent in your quest for darkness.

In addition to external factors, it's important to be mindful of the noise and light levels you create within your sleep environment. Avoid watching stimulating television shows or using electronic devices with bright screens right before bed, as these can interfere with your body's natural wind-down process. Instead, opt for relaxing activities like reading a book or practicing gentle stretching exercises to prepare your mind and body for sleep.

By taking control of the noise and light levels in your sleep environment, you can significantly improve your sleep quality and wake up feeling refreshed and rejuvenated. Experiment with different techniques until you find what works best for you. Remember, better sleep is within your reach – all it takes is a little effort and a commitment to creating a peaceful sanctuary for your slumber.

Chapter 4: Establishing a Bedtime Routine

Relaxation Techniques for Better Sleep

In today's fast-paced world, a good night's sleep is often elusive. From juggling work responsibilities to managing personal relationships, it's no wonder that so many adults struggle with getting adequate rest. However, incorporating relaxation techniques into your bedtime routine can significantly improve the quality of your sleep and leave you feeling refreshed and rejuvenated each morning.

Deep breathing exercises are a simple yet powerful technique that can help you relax before bedtime. By focusing on your breath and taking slow, deep breaths, you activate your body's natural relaxation response. This technique not only calms your mind but also reduces muscle tension, making it easier to fall asleep and stay asleep throughout the night.

Another effective relaxation technique is progressive muscle relaxation. This involves systematically tensing and then releasing each muscle group in your body, starting from your toes and working your way up to your head. By consciously focusing on the sensation of relaxation as you release each muscle group, you can effectively reduce physical tension and promote a sense of calmness conducive to better sleep.

Meditation and mindfulness practices have gained immense popularity in recent years, and for good reason. Engaging in a few minutes of meditation or mindfulness before bed can help quiet racing thoughts and calm a busy mind. By focusing on the present moment and letting go of worries and anxieties, you create a mental space that promotes relaxation and prepares your mind for a restful sleep.

Creating a soothing bedtime routine can also contribute to better sleep. Consider incorporating activities such as reading a book, taking a warm bath, or listening to soft music into your evening ritual. These activities can help signal to your body and mind that it's time to unwind and prepare for sleep.

Lastly, incorporating relaxation techniques into your daily life, beyond just before bed, can have a profound impact on your sleep quality. Engaging in regular physical exercise, practicing stress management techniques, and avoiding stimulating activities close to bedtime can all contribute to a more restful night's sleep.

Remember, improving your sleep is a journey, and it may take time to find the relaxation techniques that work best for you. Experiment with different strategies, and be patient with yourself. With consistent practice and a commitment to prioritizing your sleep, you can unlock the secrets to restful nights and wake upfeeling more energized and ready to tackle each day.

The Power of Regular Sleep Schedule

The Better Sleep Solution: Unlocking the Secrets to Restful Nights

In our fast-paced, technology-driven world, getting a good night's sleep has become increasingly challenging. However, the importance of a regular sleep schedule cannotbe overstated, as it holds the key to unlocking the secrets of restful nights. This subchapter explores the transformative power of maintaining a consistent sleep routine and offers practical tips for adults of all ages (18-80) on how to sleep better.

Our bodies have a natural internal clock, known as the circadian rhythm, which regulates our sleep-wake cycle. When we follow a regular sleep schedule, we alignourselves with this natural rhythm, allowing our bodies to function optimally.

Consistency is key; going to bed and waking up at the same time every day trains our bodies to anticipate sleep, leading to more restful nights and increased daytime alertness.

For adults, adhering to a regular sleep schedule can have a profound impact on overallwell-being. It enhances cognitive function, memory consolidation, creativity, and problem-solving abilities. Moreover, it boosts immune function, reduces the risk of chronic diseases such as obesity, diabetes, and cardiovascular issues, and improves mood and emotional stability.

Establishing a regular sleep schedule is not always easy, especially with the demands of work, family, and social commitments. However, with a few simple strategies, it is achievable. Firstly, prioritize sleep by setting aside a consistent block of time for rest. Create a relaxing bedtime routine that signals to your body that it's time to wind down. This could include activities such as reading, taking a warm bath, or practicing relaxation techniques like deep breathing or meditation.

Avoid stimulating activities, such as using electronic devices, within an hour before bed, as the blue light emitted by screens can disrupt the production of melatonin, a hormone that regulates sleep. Additionally, limit caffeine and alcohol intake, as they can interfere with sleep quality and disrupt the circadian rhythm.

If you find it challenging to fall asleep or stay asleep, consider incorporating naturalsleep aids like herbal teas, essential oils, or white noise machines into your routine.

However, if sleep problems persist, it is important to consult with a healthcareprofessional who can provide further guidance and support.

In conclusion, the power of a regular sleep schedule cannot be overstated. By aligningourselves with our natural internal clock, we can unlock the secrets to restful nights.

By prioritizing sleep, establishing a relaxing bedtime routine, and avoiding sleep-disrupting factors, adults of all ages can experience the countless benefits of a goodnight's rest. So, let's embrace the power of a regular sleep schedule and unlock the secrets to restful nights for a healthier, happier life.

Winding Down: Activities to Promote Sleep

In our fast-paced world, it's no surprise that many adults struggle to get a good night's sleep. The constant demands of work, family, and technology can leave us feeling overwhelmed and wired, making it difficult to unwind and fall asleep. However, there are numerous activities you can incorporate into your daily routine to promote better sleep and enjoy restful nights.

1. Create a Bedtime Routine: Establishing a consistent bedtime routine signals to your body that it's time to wind down. Engage in relaxing activities such as reading a book, taking a warm bath, or practicing gentle stretching exercises. Avoid stimulating activities like watching TV or using electronic devices, as the blue light emitted can disrupt your natural sleep-wake cycle.

2. Practice Mindfulness and Meditation: Incorporate mindfulness techniques into your nighttime routine to quiet your mind and promote relaxation. Deep breathing exercises or guided meditation can help release tension and prepare your body for sleep. Apps and podcasts provide a wide range of options suitable for beginners or those experienced in meditation.

3. Create a Sleep-Friendly Environment: Ensure your bedroom is a calm

and comfortable space conducive to sleep. Keep the room dark, cool, and quiet. Consider investing in blackout curtains, earplugs, or a white noise machine to block out any distractions that may disrupt your sleep.

4. Limit Caffeine and Alcohol: Avoid consuming caffeinated beverages or alcohol close to bedtime. Caffeine is a stimulant that can interfere with falling asleep, while alcohol may disrupt the quality of your sleep. Opt for herbal teas or warm milk insteadto promote relaxation.

5. Establish Regular Exercise: Engaging in regular physical activity during the day can help promote better sleep at night. However, avoid exercising too close to bedtime, as it may leave you feeling energized and make it harder to wind down.

6. Journaling: Writing down your thoughts, worries, or to-do lists before bed can helpclear your mind and reduce anxiety. This practice can promote a sense of calm and relaxation, making it easier to fall asleep.

Remember, everyone's sleep needs are unique. Experiment with different activities to find the ones that work best for you. It may take time to establish a routine, but with consistency and dedication, you can unlock the secrets to restful nights and experience the rejuvenating power of a good night's sleep.

Chapter 5: Managing Stress and Anxiety for Improved Sleep

Recognizing the Effects of Stress on Sleep

In today's fast-paced and demanding world, stress has become an inevitable part of our lives. It affects us in various ways, including our ability to get a good night's sleep. Understanding the impact of stress on sleep is crucial for adults of all ages, as quality sleep is essential for overall well-being and optimal functioning.

Stress can manifest in different forms, such as work pressure, financial worries, relationship issues, or health concerns. When we experience stress, our bodies release hormones like cortisol, which can disrupt our sleep patterns. This can lead to difficulties falling asleep, staying asleep, or even experiencing restless and unrefreshing sleep.

One of the most common effects of stress on sleep is racing thoughts. Many adults find it challenging to quiet their minds at night, as worries and anxieties tend to resurface when they finally have a moment of calm. This mental chatter can make it difficult to relax and unwind, preventing a restful night's sleep.

Stress can also cause physical discomfort, leading to muscle tension and pain. This can make it uncomfortable to find a comfortable sleeping position, resulting in tossing and turning throughout the night. Additionally, stress can contribute to the development of sleep disorders such as insomnia, sleep apnea, or restless leg syndrome, further exacerbating sleep difficulties.

Furthermore, stress can disrupt the natural sleep-wake cycle, also known as the circadian rhythm. The body's internal clock relies on consistency and routine to regulate sleep patterns. However, chronic stress can throw off this delicate balance, causing irregular sleep schedules, daytime drowsiness, and difficulties in maintaininga regular sleep routine.

Recognizing the effects of stress on sleep is the first step towards finding effective solutions to improve sleep quality. Managing stress through various relaxation techniques can significantly alleviate its impact on sleep. Incorporating practices suchas deep breathing exercises, meditation, or gentle stretching before bed can help calm the mind and relax the body, promoting a more peaceful sleep.

Additionally, creating a conducive sleep environment free from distractions and implementing a consistent sleep routine can also aid in reducing stress-related sleep disturbances. Establishing a regular bedtime routine that includes activities like reading, taking a warm bath, or listening to soothing music can signal to the body thatit's time to wind down and prepare for sleep.

In conclusion, stress has a profound effect on sleep quality, making it crucial for adultsof all ages to recognize and address its impact. By understanding how stress can disrupt sleep patterns and implementing effective stress management techniques, individuals can significantly improve their sleep and overall well-being. Prioritizing restful nights will lead to increased productivity, better mental health, and a happier, healthier life.

Stress-Reducing Techniques

In our fast-paced modern world, stress has become an all too common companion for people of all ages. From work pressures to personal responsibilities, stress can often disrupt our sleep patterns and lead to restless nights. However, there are various effective techniques that can help reduce stress and improve the quality of our sleep. In this subchapter, we will explore some proven stress-reducing techniques that can help you achieve restful nights and wake up feeling refreshed.

1. Deep Breathing Exercises: One of the simplest yet most effective stress-reducing techniques is deep breathing. By taking slow, deep breaths, you can activate the body's relaxation response, calming your mind and reducing stress levels. Try inhaling deeply through your nose, counting to four, and exhaling slowly through your mouth, counting to six. Repeat this process several times to experience its calming effects.

2. Progressive Muscle Relaxation: This technique involves systematically tensing and then relaxing each muscle group in your

body. Starting from your toes and working your way up to your head, tense each muscle group for a few seconds and then release the tension. This practice helps promote relaxation and can alleviate stress before bedtime.

3. Mindfulness Meditation: Practicing mindfulness meditation can significantly reduce stress levels and promote better sleep. By focusing your attention on the present moment and accepting it without judgment, you can cultivate a sense of calm and relaxation. Mindfulness can be achieved through various techniques such as guided meditation, body scan, or simply focusing on your breath.

4. Journaling: Writing down your thoughts and emotions in a journal can be a therapeutic practice to manage stress and improve sleep quality. Take a few minutes before bed to jot down any worries, concerns, or positive experiences from the day. This process can help you clear your mind, process your emotions, and create a sense of closure before sleep.

5. Physical Exercise: Engaging in regular physical exercise is not only beneficial for your overall health but can also help reduce stress and promote better sleep. Whether it's going for a walk, practicing yoga, or participating in aerobic activities, exercise releases endorphins, which are natural stress-busters, and can improve your sleep- wake

cycle.

By incorporating these stress-reducing techniques into your daily routine, you can create a peaceful and conducive environment for a restful night's sleep. Remember, everyone is unique, so experiment with different techniques to find what works bestfor you. With practice, you can effectively manage stress, improve your sleep quality,and wake up feeling rejuvenated.

Cognitive Behavioral Therapy for Insomnia (CBT-I)

In our modern, fast-paced world, getting a good night's sleep has become increasingly challenging for many adults. The inability to fall asleep or stay asleep can have a significant impact on our overall well-being, affecting our mood, productivity, and even our physical health. If you find yourself struggling with insomnia, Cognitive Behavioral Therapy for Insomnia (CBT-I) may hold the key to unlocking restful nights and improving your sleep quality.

CBT-I is a proven, evidence-based therapy that targets the underlying thoughts, beliefs, and behaviors that contribute to sleep problems. Unlike medication-based approaches, CBT-I addresses the root causes of insomnia, helping you to develop healthier sleep habits and beliefs that promote long-term sleep improvements.

One of the core principles of CBT-I is sleep hygiene, which involves creating a conducive sleep environment and establishing a regular sleep routine. This may include setting a consistent bedtime and wake-up time, avoiding stimulating activities close to bedtime, and creating a relaxing pre-sleep routine to signal yourbody that it's time to wind down.

Another important aspect of CBT-I is cognitive restructuring, which involves challenging and replacing negative thoughts and worries that may be keeping you awake. By learning to identify and reframe these thoughts, you can reduce anxietyand create a more peaceful mindset before bed.

CBT-I also incorporates stimulus control techniques to help strengthen the association between your bed and sleep. This may involve limiting the time youspend in bed when you're unable to sleep and using your bed only for sleep andintimacy, rather than for activities like watching TV or working.

In addition to these strategies, relaxation techniques such as deep breathing exercises, progressive muscle relaxation, or guided imagery can be employed to calmthe mind and prepare the body for sleep.

While CBT-I is typically administered by a trained therapist, there are also self-help resources available, including books, online programs, and mobile applications that can guide you through the process. However, it's important to note that for more severe or chronic insomnia, seeking professional help is recommended to ensure the best results.

By incorporating CBT-I techniques into your life, you can take control of your sleepand achieve the restful nights you deserve. Remember, better sleep leads to improved overall well-being, increased productivity, and a happier, healthier you. Sowhy wait? Unlock the secrets to restful nights and start your journey towards better sleep today.

Chapter 6: Enhancing Sleep Quality Through Lifestyle Changes

Exercise and Its Impact on Sleep

Introduction:

In today's fast-paced world, many adults struggle to achieve a restful night's sleep. With the increasing demands of work, family, and personal responsibilities, it can be challenging to find time for quality rest. However, one powerful tool that can significantly improve your sleep is exercise. Regular physical activity not only benefits your overall health but also has a profound impact on the quality and duration of your sleep.

The Connection between Exercise and Sleep:

Engaging in regular exercise has been proven to promote better sleep. When you exert yourself physically, your body releases endorphins, which are natural mood boosters that can reduce stress and anxiety. As a result, your mind becomes more relaxed, allowing you to fall asleep faster and experience deeper, more restorative sleep.

Exercise also helps regulate your body's internal clock, known as the circadian rhythm.

By exposing yourself to natural light during outdoor activities, your body becomes more synchronized with the day-night cycle, making it easier to fall asleep at nightand wake up in the morning.

The Timing and Type of Exercise:

To optimize the impact of exercise on your sleep, it is crucial to consider the timing and type of physical activity. Engaging in vigorous exercise close to bedtime can lead to increased alertness, making it difficult to fall asleep. Therefore, it is recommended to finish your workout at least two to three hours before bedtime.

The best types of exercise for improving sleep include aerobic activities, such as walking, jogging, cycling, or swimming. These exercises elevate your heart rate and body temperature, stimulating the release of endorphins. However, strength training and yoga can also be beneficial as they promote muscle relaxation and reduce tension, contributing to a more restful sleep.

Creating a Balanced Exercise Routine:

It is essential to strike a balance between exercise and rest to optimize your sleepquality. Overtraining or pushing your body beyond its limits can lead to increased stress and difficulty sleeping. Therefore, it is crucial to listen to your body's cues and avoid excessive exercise, especially if you experience fatigue or pain.

Conclusion:

Exercise is a powerful tool that can significantly improve your sleep. By incorporating regular physical activity into your daily routine, you can reap the benefits of reduced stress, improved mood, and better sleep quality. Remember to choose the right timing and type of exercise that suits your lifestyle and preferences, allowing you to unlock the secrets to restful nights and experience the rejuvenating power of a good night's sleep.

Dietary Habits for Optimal Sleep

Introduction:

In our quest for a good night's sleep, we often overlook the role that our dietary habits play in promoting restful nights. What we eat and drink throughout the day can significantly impact the quality and duration of our sleep. By adopting a few dietary habits, you can optimize your sleep and wake up feeling refreshed and energized. In this subchapter, we will delve into the various ways in which your diet can positively influence your sleep patterns.

1. Avoid Stimulants:

First and foremost, it's crucial to limit the consumption of stimulants such as caffeine and nicotine, especially in the hours leading up to bedtime. These substances can interfere with your ability to fall asleep and stay asleep, disrupting your natural sleep- wake cycle. Instead, opt for herbal teas or warm milk, which contain sleep-promoting compounds like chamomile or tryptophan.

2.   Promote Serotonin Production:

Foods rich in tryptophan, an amino acid that aids in the production of serotonin, can help regulate sleep patterns. Incorporate sources of tryptophan into your diet, such asturkey, chicken, bananas, nuts, and seeds. Serotonin, a neurotransmitter, promotes relaxation and helps regulate mood and sleep.

3.   Magnesium and Melatonin:

Magnesium and melatonin are two essential compounds that contribute to healthy sleep. Magnesium-rich foods like leafy greens, nuts, and legumes can help relax muscles and calm the nervous system. Additionally, melatonin, a hormone responsible for regulating sleep-wake cycles, can be found in foods like tart cherries,almonds, and oats.

4.   Avoid Heavy Meals and Spicy Foods:

Consuming heavy meals or spicy foods close to bedtime can lead to indigestion, heartburn, and discomfort, making it harder to fall asleep. Aim to have your last mealat least two to three hours before bedtime and opt for lighter, easily digestible options.

5.   Hydration and Alcohol:

Staying hydrated throughout the day is vital for overall health, including sleep quality. However, avoid excessive fluid intake close to bedtime to minimize the need for frequent trips to the bathroom during the night. Additionally, while alcohol may initially make you feel drowsy, it can disrupt the later stages of sleep, leading to a lessrestorative rest.

Conclusion:

By incorporating these dietary habits into your routine, you can optimize your sleep and reap the benefits of restful nights. Remember, making small changes to your diet can have a significant impact on your sleep quality, allowing you to wake up feeling refreshed, rejuvenated, and ready to take on the day. Sweet dreams!

Limiting Caffeine and Alcohol

In today's fast-paced world, adults of all ages find it increasingly challenging to get a good night's sleep. One major factor that affects our sleep quality is our consumption of caffeine and alcohol. These substances, often used as a means to relax or stay awake, can actually disrupt our natural sleep patterns and leave us feeling groggy and restless.

Caffeine, found in coffee, tea, energy drinks, and even some chocolate, is a stimulantthat keeps us awake and alert. While it can be a great way to kick-start your day, consuming caffeine too close to bedtime can have detrimental effects on your sleep. As a general rule, it's best to avoid caffeine at least six hours before bedtime. This allows your body enough time to metabolize the caffeine, reducing its impact on your sleep. By limiting your caffeine intake, you'll find that you fall asleep more easily and experience more restful nights.

Similarly, alcohol, often used as a way to wind down and relax, can actually disrupt our sleep cycles. While alcohol may initially make you feel drowsy and help you fall asleep faster, it can cause fragmented sleep and frequent awakenings throughout the night. These interruptions prevent you from reaching the deep, restorative stages of sleep and can leave you feeling tired and groggy the next day. If you enjoy a drink in the evening, try to finish it at least two to three hours before bedtime to give your body enough time to process the alcohol and minimize its effects on your sleep.

Instead of relying on caffeine or alcohol to manage your sleep, consider adopting healthier habits to improve your sleep quality. Engaging in regular exercise, creating a calming bedtime routine, and establishing a consistent sleep schedule are all effective strategies for achieving restful nights. Additionally, incorporating relaxation techniques like deep breathing exercises or meditation can help calm your mind and prepare your body for sleep.

In conclusion, if you're struggling to get a good night's sleep, limiting your consumption of caffeine and alcohol can greatly improve your sleep quality. By being mindful of when and how much you consume, you'll be able to establish healthier sleep habits that will leave you feeling more refreshed and rejuvenated each morning. Remember, a restful night's sleep is within your reach, and making small adjustments to your lifestyle can make a world of difference.

Chapter 7: Technological Solutions for Better Sleep

Sleep Tracking Devices and Apps

In this digital age, technology has permeated every aspect of our lives, including our sleep. Sleep tracking devices and apps has gained immense popularity as tools to help us understand and improve our sleep patterns. With their ability to monitor andanalyze our sleep quality, these devices have become indispensable for adults seeking to achieve restful nights.

Sleep tracking devices come in various forms, from wearable bands to smart watchesand even smartphone apps. They utilize advanced sensors to collect data on your sleep patterns, including duration, movement, and heart rate. By tracking these metrics, you can gain valuable insights into your sleep quality and identify potential issues that may be hindering your ability to achieve a restful night's sleep.

One of the significant benefits of sleep tracking devices and apps is their ability to provide personalized recommendations. Using the data they collect, these tools can offer tailored suggestions to improve your sleep hygiene. For example, if you notice that your sleep quality is compromised when you consume caffeine late in the day, the app might recommend cutting back on caffeine intake after a certain time. By following these suggestions, you can gradually optimize your sleep routine and experience more restorative sleep.

Another advantage of sleep tracking devices and apps is their ability to track sleep trends over time. By providing detailed sleep reports and graphs, these tools allow you to identify patterns and trends in your sleep habits. This information can be invaluable in understanding the factors that affect your sleep positively or negatively.

Armed with this knowledge, you can make informed decisions and take proactivesteps to improve your sleep quality.

It is important to note that while sleep tracking devices and apps can be incrediblyuseful, they should not replace professional medical advice. If you consistently struggle with sleep issues or suspect an underlying sleep disorder, it is crucial to consult a healthcare professional who can provide a comprehensive evaluation.

In conclusion, sleeps tracking devices and apps have revolutionized the way we understand and optimize our sleep. By utilizing their advanced technology, we cangain insights into our sleep patterns, receive personalized recommendations, and track trends over time. However, it is essential to remember that they should supplement, not replace, professional medical advice. With the help of these tools and guidance from healthcare professionals, adults of all ages can unlock the secretsto restful nights and enjoy the multitude of benefits that come with rejuvenating sleep.

White Noise Machines and Sound Therapy

The Better Sleep Solution: Unlocking the Secrets to Restful Nights

In our quest for a good night's sleep, we often overlook the importance of creating a peaceful sleeping environment. This subchapter explores the benefits of white noise machines and sound therapy, two powerful tools that can help adults of all ages sleepbetter and wake up feeling refreshed.

White noise machines have gained popularity in recent years, and for good reason. These devices emit a consistent sound that masks other noises in the environment, creating a soothing background noise that promotes relaxation and better sleep.

Whether you live in a noisy urban area or share a bedroom with a snoring partner, a white noise machine can provide the tranquility you need to drift off into a deep slumber. By drowning out disruptive sounds, these machines help you maintain a steady sleep state, reducing the likelihood of being awakened throughout the night.

On the other hand, sound therapy takes a different approach to improve sleep quality. It utilizes specific sounds and frequencies to induce a state of relaxation and promote better sleep. Various forms of sound therapy exist, such as nature sounds, binaural beats, and soothing music. These auditory stimuli can have a profound effect on our brainwaves, helping us transition into a more peaceful sleep state. For example, listening to gentle ocean waves or rainforest sounds can transport us to a serene setting, calming our mind and preparing us for a restful night's sleep.

Both white noise machines and sound therapy offer unique benefits, and the choice between the two ultimately depends on individual preferences. Some individuals find the consistent hum of white noise machines comforting, while others prefer the therapeutic effects of specific sounds. Experimenting with both options can help you discover the perfect solution for your sleep needs.

To incorporate white noise machines or sound therapy into your sleep routine,consider placing the machine near your bed or using headphones for a more immersive experience. It's important to note that these tools are not a cure-all for sleep problems, but rather a complementary approach to creating a conducive sleepenvironment.

In conclusion, white noise machines and sound therapy can be valuable allies in thequest for better sleep. By blocking out external disturbances and promoting relaxation, these tools help adults of all ages achieve restful nights. Whether you optfor the steady hum of a white noise machine or the soothing sounds of nature, incorporating these techniques into your sleep routine can unlock the secrets to atruly restorative slumber.

Blue Light Filtering and Screen Time Reduction

In today's modern world, we are constantly surrounded by screens computers, smartphones, tablets, televisions - you name it. While these devices have undoubtedly made our lives more convenient and connected, they may also be wreaking havoc on our sleep patterns. The culprit? Blue light.

Blue light is a short wavelength light emitted by natural light as well as electronic devices and energy-efficient light bulbs. It has been proven to suppress the production of melatonin, a hormone that regulates our sleep-wake cycle. This means that excessive exposure to blue light in the evening can disrupt our natural sleep patterns, making it harder to fall asleep and stay asleep throughout the night.

So, what can we do to combat the negative effects of blue light? Enter blue light filtering and screen time reduction techniques, which can help us achieve a restful night's sleep.

One effective method is to invest in blue light filtering glasses such as those offered by Sleep ZM (www.sleepzm.com) or screen protectors. These specialized lenses or filters can block or reduce the amount of blue light emitted by screens, thus minimizing its impact on our sleep. By wearing these glasses or using these filters in the evening, we can allow our bodies to naturally produce melatonin and prepare for a good night's sleep.

However, reducing screen time altogether is equally important. The constant exposure to screens, especially in the hours leading up to bedtime, can overstimulated our brains and make it difficult to unwind and relax. Consider implementing a "screen curfew" at least one hour before you plan to sleep. Instead of scrolling through social media or binge-watching your favorite TV show, engage in activities that promote relaxation, such as reading a book, practicing meditation or yoga, or taking a warmbath.

Additionally, it's crucial to create a sleep-friendly environment in your bedroom. Ensure that the lighting is dim and warm, and avoid using electronic devices in bed.

Instead, opt for a traditional alarm clock, and keep your bedroom a screen-free zone.

By making these small adjustments, you can create a peaceful and conduciveatmosphere that promotes better sleep.

In conclusion, blue light filtering and screen time reduction are essential strategies for improving the quality of our sleep. By being mindful of the amount of blue light we expose ourselves to and implementing screen-free routines before bed, we can unlock the secrets to restful nights. So, let's prioritize our sleep and reap the benefits of waking up refreshed and rejuvenated each morning.

Chapter 8: Natural Remedies and Sleep Aids

Herbal Supplements for Sleep Support

In today's fast-paced world, getting a good night's sleep can be challenging. The constant stress, busy schedules, and endless distractions can wreak havoc on our sleep patterns, leaving us feeling tired and groggy during the day. Fortunately, there are natural remedies available to help support healthy sleep, and herbal supplementscan play a key role in achieving restful nights.

One of the most popular herbal supplements for sleep support is valerian root.

Valerian has been used for centuries as a natural sleep aid due to its calming properties. It works by increasing the levels of a neurotransmitter called gamma-amino butyric acid (GABA) in the brain, which helps to calm the nervous system and promote relaxation. Studies have shown that valerian root can improve sleep quality, reduce the time it takes to fall asleep, and decrease nighttime awakenings.

Another powerful herbal supplement is chamomile. Known for its soothing properties,chamomile tea has long been used as a bedtime ritual to promote relaxation and sleep. Chamomile contains apigenin, a compound that binds to specific receptors inthe brain, reducing anxiety and promoting sleepiness.

Consuming chamomile tea before bedtime can help calm the mind and prepare the body for a restful night's sleep.

Passionflower is another herbal supplement that has been used for centuries as a natural sleep aid. It works by increasing the levels of GABA in the brain, similar to valerian root. Passionflower has been found to improve sleep quality, reduce anxiety,and enhance overall relaxation. It is particularly effective for those experiencing insomnia related to anxiety and racing thoughts.

Lastly, melatonin is a hormone naturally produced by the body that regulates sleep- wake cycles. However, many adults may have imbalances in melatonin production, leading to difficulty falling asleep or staying asleep. Taking a melatonin supplement can help regulate these sleep-wake cycles, making it easier to fall asleep and improving overall sleep quality.

While herbal supplements can be effective in supporting healthy sleep, it's important to consult with a healthcare professional before starting any new regimen, especially if you have any underlying health conditions or are taking other medications.

Additionally, it's crucial to prioritize good sleep hygiene practices such as maintaining a consistent sleep schedule, creating a relaxing bedtime routine, and creating a sleep-friendly environment.

In conclusion, herbal supplements can be a valuable addition to any sleep supportregimen. Valerian root, chamomile, passionflower, and melatonin are all natural remedies that have been shown to improve sleep quality and promote relaxation. However, it's important to remember that everyone's sleep needs are different, and what works for one person may not work for another. By exploring different herbal supplements and finding the right combination for your individual needs, you can unlock the secrets to restful nights and wake up feeling refreshed and rejuvenatedeach day.

Aromatherapy and Essential Oils

In our modern, fast-paced world, achieving a good night's sleep can often seem like an elusive goal. The constant stress and endless thoughts swirling in our minds can make it challenging to unwind and relax when it's time to sleep. However, there is a natural and effective solution that has been used for centuries to promote restful nights - aromatherapy and essential oils.

Aromatherapy is a holistic healing practice that utilizes the power of scent to enhancephysical and mental well-being. Essential oils, derived from plant extracts, are the primary tools used in aromatherapy. These oils contain potent aromatic compoundsthat can positively impact our mood, emotions, and overall sleep quality.

One of the most popular essential oils for sleep is lavender. Known for its calming and soothing properties, lavender oil can help alleviate anxiety and stress, promoting a sense of relaxation. Diffusing a few drops of lavender oil in your bedroom before sleep can create a tranquil environment, conducive to a restful night.

Another essential oil renowned for its sleep-inducing effects is chamomile. This gentle and mild oil can help reduce insomnia and promote deep sleep. Applying a few drops of chamomile oil to your pillow or adding it to a warm bath before bedtime can help you unwind and prepare your body for a peaceful slumber.

If you struggle with sleep disturbances caused by congestion or respiratory issues, eucalyptus oil might be your go-to choice. This invigorating oil can clear nasal passages, ease breathing, and enhance overall sleep quality. A few drops of eucalyptus oil added to a diffuser or a hot steamy shower can provide relief and improve your ability to sleep soundly.

In addition to these essential oils, there are numerous other options to explore, such as bergamot, ylang-ylang, and sandalwood, each with its unique properties to support better sleep. However, it is important to note that essential oils should be used with caution. Always dilute them properly and consult a professional if you have any existing health conditions or are pregnant.

By incorporating aromatherapy and essential oils into your sleep routine, you can create a peaceful and inviting atmosphere that promotes relaxation and restful nights. Experiment with different scents and find what works best for you. Remember, a good night's sleep is within reach, and with the power of aromatherapy, you can unlock the secrets to a rejuvenating slumber.

Melatonin and Other Sleep Aids

In our fast-paced modern lives, it is not uncommon for adults of all ages to struggle with getting a good night's sleep. The relentless demands of work, family, and other responsibilities often leave us feeling frazzled and unable to unwind when it's time to sleep. Fortunately, there are various sleep aids available that can help us achieve the restful nights we desperately need. One such aid is melatonin, a hormone produced naturally by the body to regulate our sleep-wake cycles.

Melatonin supplements have gained popularity in recent years, and for good reason. They can be an effective tool in helping us fall asleep faster and stay asleep longer. Melatonin is particularly beneficial for those who have trouble falling asleep due to jet lag, shift work, or other disruptions to their sleep schedule. It can also be helpful for individuals with certain sleep disorders, such as insomnia.

As we discussed earlier, blue light blocking glasses such as those offered by Sleep ZM (www.sleepzm.com) can help you to block blue light and let your body produce Melatonin on its own. However, it is important to note that melatonin is not a cure-all for sleep problems. While it can be a useful supplement, it should not be relied upon as a long-term solution. It is always best to address the underlying factors contributing to poor sleep, such as stress, anxiety, or poor sleep hygiene.

In addition to melatonin, there are other sleep aids available on the market. These include over-the-counter medications, herbal remedies, and relaxation techniques. It is crucial to consult with a healthcare professional before trying any sleep aid, as they can help determine the best course of action based on your individual needs and health conditions.

Furthermore, it is essential to understand that sleep aids should only be used as a temporary solution. Developing healthy sleep habits and a bedtime routine that promotes relaxation and restfulness is key to achieving long-term sleep improvement. This may include creating a sleep-friendly environment, limiting exposure to electronic devices before bed, and practicing relaxation techniques suchas deep breathing or meditation.

In conclusion, melatonin and other sleep aids can be beneficial tools in achieving better sleep, especially for those with specific sleep challenges. However, it is essential to approach these aids with caution and consult with a healthcare professional. Ultimately, the path to restful nights lies in developing healthy sleep habits and addressing the root causes of sleep disturbances. By prioritizing sleep and implementing effective strategies, adults of all ages can unlock the secrets to a trulyrestorative night's rest.

Chapter 9: Seeking Professional Help for Persistent Sleep Issues

When to Consult a Sleep Specialist

Sleep is an essential part of our lives, impacting our physical and mental well-being in profound ways. However, for many adults, achieving restful nights can be a challenge. If you find yourself struggling with sleep issues despite trying various remedies, it may be time to consult a sleep specialist. These experts are highly trained in diagnosing and treating sleep disorders, providing invaluable guidance to help you achieve the sleep you deserve.

One common misconception is that sleep problems are merely a normal part of life or a result of stress. While stress can indeed impact sleep, chronic sleep disturbances should not be ignored. If you regularly experience difficulties falling asleep, staying asleep, or waking up feeling tired despite adequate hours of sleep, it is crucial to seek professional advice.

A sleep specialist can help identify the underlying causes of your sleep issues. They will conduct a comprehensive evaluation, which may include a detailed medical history, a physical examination, and possibly even a sleep study. This study involves monitoring your sleep patterns, brain activity, and body movements to pinpoint any abnormalities or disorders such as sleep apnea, insomnia, or restless leg syndrome.

Consulting a sleep specialist is particularly important if you experience other symptoms alongside your sleep problems. These symptoms could include loud snoring, gasping or choking during sleep, excessive daytime sleepiness, sudden leg movements, or frequent nightmares. Such signs may indicate the presence of a sleepdisorder that requires medical intervention.

Furthermore, certain medical conditions such as diabetes, heart disease, or depressioncan significantly impact sleep quality. If you have been diagnosed with any of these conditions and find that they are interfering with your ability to sleep well, a sleep specialist can work in conjunction with your primary care physician to develop a comprehensive treatment plan.

Remember, sleep is not a luxury but a necessity for optimal health and well-being. Byconsulting a sleep specialist, you are taking a proactive step towards addressing your sleep concerns and improving your quality of life. Don't suffer in silence; reach out to a sleep specialist today and unlock the secrets to restful nights.

Diagnostic Tests for Sleep Disorders

In order to address the issue of sleep disorders and help individuals achieve restful nights, it is crucial to understand the diagnostic tests available to accurately identify and treat these conditions. Diagnostic tests for sleep disorders play a vital role in determining the underlying causes and severity of sleep disturbances. This subchapter aims to familiarize adults aged 18-80, seeking to improve their sleep quality, with the various diagnostic tests used in sleep medicine.

Polysomnography (PSG) is one of the most comprehensive diagnostic tests for sleep disorders. This non-invasive test involves monitoring brain waves, eye movements, muscle activity, heart rate, and breathing patterns while an individual sleeps. PSG helps identify disorders such as sleep apnea, narcolepsy, and periodic limb movementdisorder, among others.

Another useful diagnostic test is the Multiple Sleep Latency Test (MSLT). This test measures daytime sleepiness and helps diagnose conditions such as narcolepsy. It involves multiple nap opportunities throughout the day, during which the time taken to fall asleep is measured. This test provides valuable insights into an individual's daytime sleepiness and sleep-wake patterns.

Actigraphy is a diagnostic test that involves wearing a wristwatch-like device that records movement and light exposure. This test is particularly useful in assessing circadian rhythm disorders and can provide valuable information on an individual'ssleep patterns over an extended period.

Additionally, the Epworth Sleepiness Scale (ESS) is a questionnaire-based diagnostic tool that measures an individual's daytime sleepiness. By rating the likelihood of dozing off in various situations, the ESS helps identify excessive daytime sleepiness,a common symptom of several sleep disorders.

Furthermore, a comprehensive sleep evaluation may involve additional tests such as the maintenance of wakefulness test (MWT) to assess alertness during the day, the Berlin Questionnaire to screen for sleep apnea risk, or a home sleep apnea test (HSAT) for a more convenient evaluation of sleep apnea.

Understanding the available diagnostic tests for sleep disorders is critical for adults seeking to improve their sleep quality. By identifying the underlying causes and severity of sleep disturbances, these tests pave the way for effective treatment strategies and ultimately lead to restful nights and improved overall well-being. If you are struggling with sleep issues, it is advisable to consult a sleep specialist who can guide you through the diagnostic process and help you find the most appropriate solutions for your specific sleep concerns.

Treatment Options for Chronic Sleep Problems

When it comes to chronic sleep problems, finding effective treatment options is crucial for adults of all ages. Lack of quality sleep can lead to a variety of health issues, including increased stress levels, impaired cognitive function, and a weakened immune system. In this subchapter, we will explore some of the most effective treatments for chronic sleep problems, providing you with the tools to achieve restful nights and improved overall well-being.

The Better Sleep Solution: Unlocking the Secrets to Restful Nights

1. Cognitive-Behavioral Therapy for Insomnia (CBT-I): One of the most recommended treatments for chronic sleep problems is CBT-I. This therapy focuses on identifying and changing negative thoughts and behaviors that contribute to sleep difficulties. By working with a trained therapist, you can learn relaxation techniques, establish a consistent sleep schedule, and develop effective strategies to manage stress and anxiety.

2. Medications: In some cases, medications may be prescribed to help manage chronic sleep problems. However, it is important to consult with a healthcare professional before starting any medication regimen. They will evaluate your specific needs and determine if medications, such as sleep aids or anti-anxiety medications are appropriate for your situation.

3. Sleep Hygiene Practices: Implementing good sleep hygiene practices can significantly improve your sleep quality. This includes creating a relaxing bedtime routine, keeping a consistent sleep schedule, avoiding stimulants like caffeine and nicotine before bed, and creating a comfortable sleep environment free from distractions.

4. Relaxation Techniques: Incorporating relaxation techniques into your daily routine can help prepare your body and mind for sleep. Deep breathing exercises, progressive muscle relaxation, and mindfulness meditation are examples of techniques that can calm your mind and promote relaxation.

5. Alternative Therapies: Some individuals find relief from chronic sleep problems through alternative therapies such as acupuncture, aromatherapy, or herbal supplements. While the effectiveness of these treatments varies from person to person, it may be worth exploring these options in conjunction with other evidence-based treatments.

Remember, treating chronic sleep problems requires a multifaceted approach tailored to your specific needs. It is essential to consult with a healthcare professional who can evaluate your situation, provide personalized recommendations, and monitor your progress. By taking proactive steps towards improving your sleep, you can unlock the secrets to restful nights and enjoy better overall health and well-being.

Chapter 10: Maintaining Healthy Sleep Habits in the Long Run

Overcoming Common Sleep Challenges

Sleep is an essential part of our daily routine, yet many adults struggle to achieve a restful night's sleep. Whether it's difficulty falling asleep, waking up frequently duringthe night, or feeling exhausted even after a full night's rest, these common sleep challenges can greatly impact our overall well-being. However, with the right strategies and adjustments, it is possible to overcome these obstacles and unlock thesecrets to restful nights.

One of the most common sleep challenges is insomnia, which can manifest as difficulty falling asleep, staying asleep, or waking up too early. To combat insomnia, it is important to establish a consistent sleep routine. Going to bed and waking up at the same time every day helps regulate the body's internal clock and signals it when it's time to sleep. Additionally, creating a relaxing bedtime routine, such as reading a bookor taking a warm bath, can help signal the body to wind down and prepare for sleep.

Another common sleep challenge is sleep apnea, a condition characterized by interrupted breathing during sleep. Sleep apnea often goes undiagnosed, yet it can significantly impact the quality of sleep. If you suspect you may have sleep apnea, it is crucial to consult a healthcare professional who can provide a proper diagnosis and recommend appropriate treatment options such as continuous positive airway pressure (CPAP) therapy.

Stress and anxiety can also disrupt sleep patterns, leading to restless nights. To combat these challenges, it is important to engage in stress-reducing activities before bed. This may include deep breathing exercises, meditation, or journaling to clear the mind of any worries or racing thoughts. Creating a peaceful sleep environment by minimizing noise, reducing light, and ensuring a comfortable temperature can also contribute to a more restful sleep.

Lastly, technology can be a significant hindrance to achieving a restful night's sleep.

The blue light emitted by electronic devices such as smartphones, tablets, and laptops can interfere with the body's production of melatonin, a hormone that regulates sleep. It is advisable to limit the use of electronic devices at least an hour before bed and create a technology-free zone in the bedroom.

By implementing these strategies and making necessary adjustments, adults of all ages can overcome common sleep challenges and improve their ability to sleep better. Remember, sleep is not a luxury but a fundamental necessity for overall health and well-being. With a commitment to better sleep hygiene, you can unlock the secrets to restful nights and wake up feeling refreshed and rejuvenated each day.

Tips for Traveling and Adjusting to New Time Zones

Traveling to different time zones can be exciting and adventurous, but it can also disrupt your sleep patterns and leave you feeling exhausted. Whether you're a frequent traveler or embarking on a once-in-a-lifetime trip, it's essential to know how to adjust to new time zones and ensure you get a restful night's sleep. Here are some helpful tips to help you sleep better and adapt to different time zones seamlessly.

1. Plan ahead: Before your trip, gradually adjust your sleeping schedule to align with the time zone of your destination. This means going to bed earlier or later, depending on the time difference. Start adjusting your sleep schedule a few days before your trip to minimize jet lag and help your body adapt more easily.

2. Stay hydrated: Drinking plenty of water during your flight can help combat the dehydrating effects of air travel and keep you feeling refreshed. Avoid excessive caffeine and alcohol, as they can disrupt your sleep patterns and worsen jet lag symptoms.

3. Optimize your sleep environment: Create a sleep-friendly environment wherever you go. Pack an eye mask, earplugs, and a travel-sized pillow to ensure you can sleep comfortably in unfamiliar surroundings. If you're sensitive to light, consider using blackout curtains or a sleep mask to block out any unwanted light.

4. Get natural light exposure: Upon arrival at your destination, expose yourself to natural sunlight as much as possible. Natural light helps regulate your internal body clock and signals to your brain that it's time to be awake. Spend time outside duringdaylight hours to help your body adjust to the new time zone.

5. Stick to a routine: Establishing a consistent sleep routine while traveling can help your body adjust more quickly. Try to go to bed and wake up at the same time each day, even if it means adjusting your schedule temporarily. This consistency will signal your body when it's time to sleep and when it's time to wake up.

6. Consider short-term sleep aids: If you're struggling to adjust to a new time zone, consider using short-term sleep aids such as melatonin. Melatonin is a hormone that regulates sleep-wake cycles and can help reset your internal clock. Consult with a healthcare professional before using any sleep aids to ensure they are safe for you.

By following these tips, you can minimize the effects of jet lag and ensure a restful night's sleep while traveling. Remember, adjusting to a new time zone takes time, so be patient with yourself and give your body the time it needs to adapt. With a little preparation and a mindful approach, you can make the most of your travels while maintaining a healthy sleep routine.

Sleep Hygiene Maintenance for Lifelong Benefits

Sleep is a fundamental aspect of our overall health and well-being. It plays a crucial role in our physical, mental, and emotional functioning. Unfortunately, many adults struggle with achieving restful nights, leading to a variety of negative consequences in their daily lives. However, by implementing proper sleep hygiene maintenance techniques, you can improve your sleep quality and reap the lifelong benefits it offers.

Establishing a consistent sleep schedule is paramount in optimizing your sleep hygiene. Aim to go to bed and wake up at the same time every day, even on weekends. This helps regulate your body's internal clock and promotes a natural sleep-wake cycle. Additionally, create a relaxing bedtime routine that signals to your body that it's time to wind down. This can include activities like reading a book, taking a warm bath, or practicing relaxation techniques such as deep breathing or meditation.

Creating a sleep-friendly environment is another vital aspect of sleep hygiene maintenance. Ensure your bedroom is cool, dark, and quiet. Invest in a comfortable mattress and pillows that support your body's needs. Limit exposure to electronic devices before bed, as the blue light emitted can disrupt your sleep patterns. Consider using blackout curtains, earplugs, or a white noise machine to further enhance your sleep environment.

Your daytime habits also significantly impact your sleep quality. Engaging in regular physical activity can promote better sleep, but avoid exercising too close to bedtime, as it may energize you. Be mindful of your caffeine and alcohol intake, as they can interfere with your ability to fall asleep or stay asleep. It's essential to strike a balance.

Managing stress and anxiety is crucial for achieving restful nights. Incorporate stress- reducing activities into your daily routine, such as journaling, practicing mindfulness, or engaging in hobbies you enjoy. If you find it challenging to quiet your mind at night, consider implementing relaxation techniques like progressive muscle relaxationor guided imagery.

By prioritizing sleep hygiene maintenance, you can experience a myriad of lifelong benefits. Improved sleep quality leads to enhanced cognitive function, increased productivity, better mood regulation, and a reduced risk of chronic health conditionssuch as heart disease and obesity. Take the necessary steps today to unlock the secrets of restful nights and enjoy the countless advantages that come with it.

Conclusion: Embracing the Sleep Solution for Restful Nights

In this book, "The Sleep Solution: Unlocking the Secrets to Restful Nights," we havedelved into the world of sleep and explored how to improve the quality of your rest. Now, as we reach the conclusion, it is time to summarize the key takeaways and encourage you to embrace the sleep solution for restful nights.

Sleep is an essential aspect of our lives, impacting our physical and mental well- being. Unfortunately, many adults today struggle with sleep issues, ranging from difficulty falling asleep to waking up multiple times during the night. However, the good news is that there are effective strategies and techniques that can help you sleep better.

Throughout this book, we have covered various aspects of sleep, including the importance of establishing a consistent sleep schedule, creating a sleep-friendly environment, and adopting relaxation techniques to calm your mind before bed. We have also discussed the impact of lifestyle factors such as diet, exercise, and technology on sleep quality.

One of the key takeaways from this book is the significance of prioritizing sleep.

Often, in our busy lives, we tend to neglect sleep and prioritize other tasks. However, by understanding the importance of sleep and its role in overall health, we can make conscious choices to ensure we get the rest we need.

Another crucial aspect we explored is the power of routine. Establishing a consistent sleep schedule, including waking up and going to bed at the same time every day, can train your body to recognize patterns and promote better sleep. Implementing a bedtime routine that includes relaxation exercises like deep breathing, meditation, or reading can signal to your body that it is time to wind down and prepare for sleep.

Additionally, we discussed the impact of technology on sleep quality. The blue light emitted by electronic devices can disrupt your circadian rhythm, making it harder to fall asleep. Implementing a digital detox before bed, such as avoiding screens for at least an hour before sleep, can significantly improve your sleep.

In conclusion, by embracing the sleep solution outlined in this book, you can unlock the secrets to restful nights. From establishing a consistent sleep schedule to creating a sleep-friendly environment and prioritizing relaxation, there are numerous strategies you can implement to improve your sleep quality. Remember, sleep is not a luxury but a necessity for your overall well-being. So, take the knowledge and tools provided in this book and start your journey towards restful nights and rejuvenated days. Sweet dreams!

Sleep   ZM
Blue Light Glasses

I created Sleep ZM to help the billions of people around the world enjoy an affordable, natural way to enjoy better sleep at night, as well as avoid the myriad of painful effects caused by harmful blue light such as eyestrain, headaches, and migraines.

Like you, I sometimes had trouble falling asleep at night, so after considerable research I discovered blue light blocking glasses. After purchasing a number of topbrands, I didn't find one that met all my needs, so I decided to create my own brand and the rest is history...Sleep ZM was born, because its about time...time to sleep

Search through our blue light blocking glasses and sunglasses collections and come back often as we are always launching new products to help you sleep better...feel better...live better.

Jeff Smith